PREGNANCY COLORING BOOK

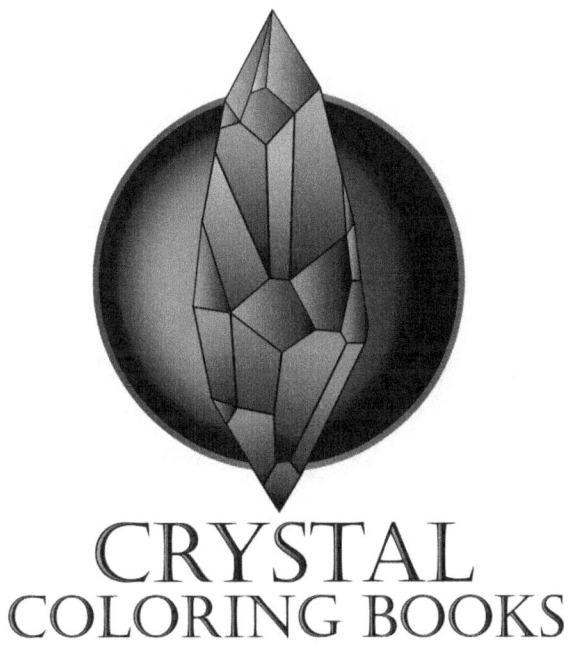

CRYSTAL
COLORING BOOKS

Copyright © 2018 Crystal Coloring Books
All rights reserved.
ISBN-13: 978-1986600439
ISBN-10: 1986600432

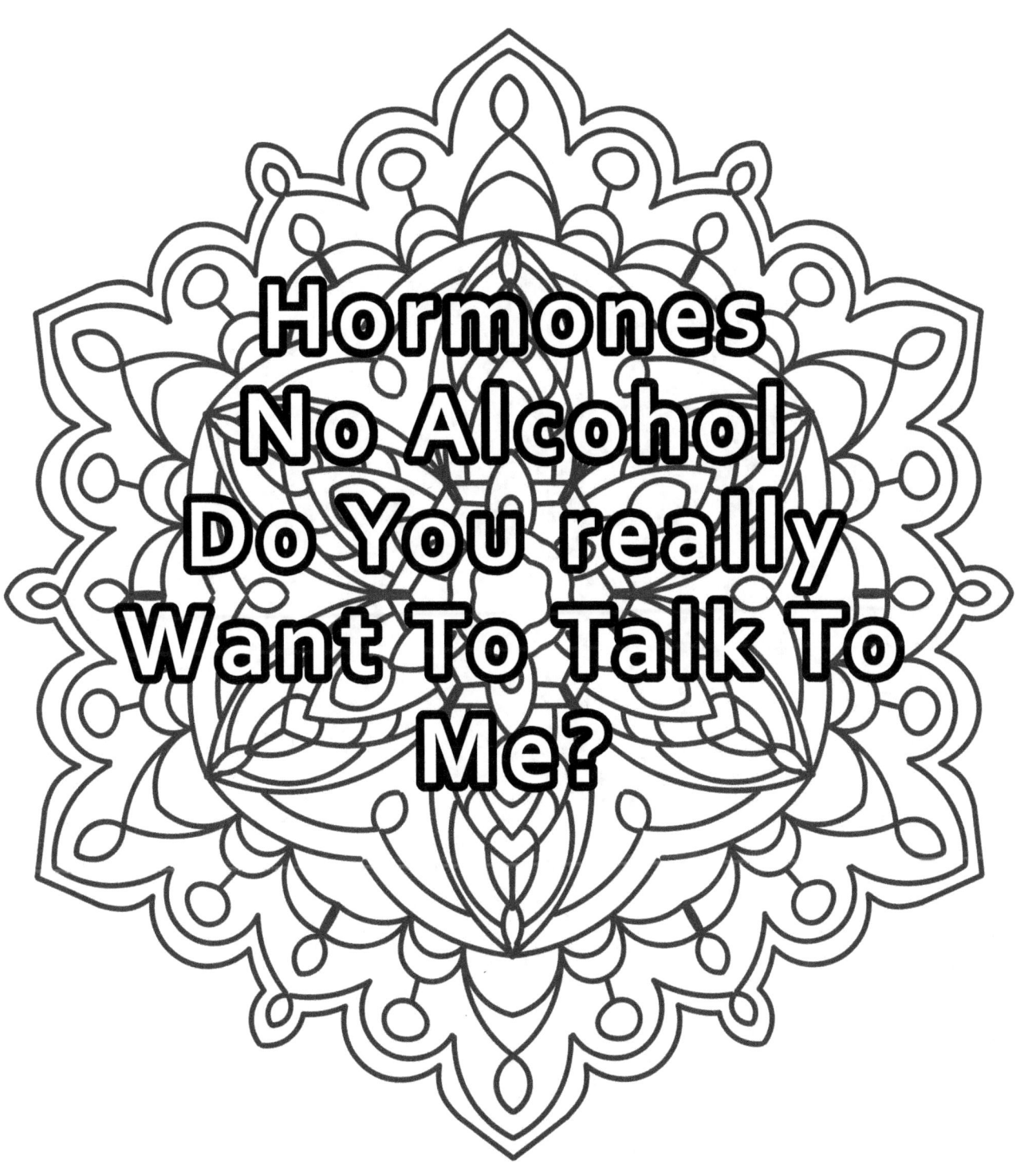

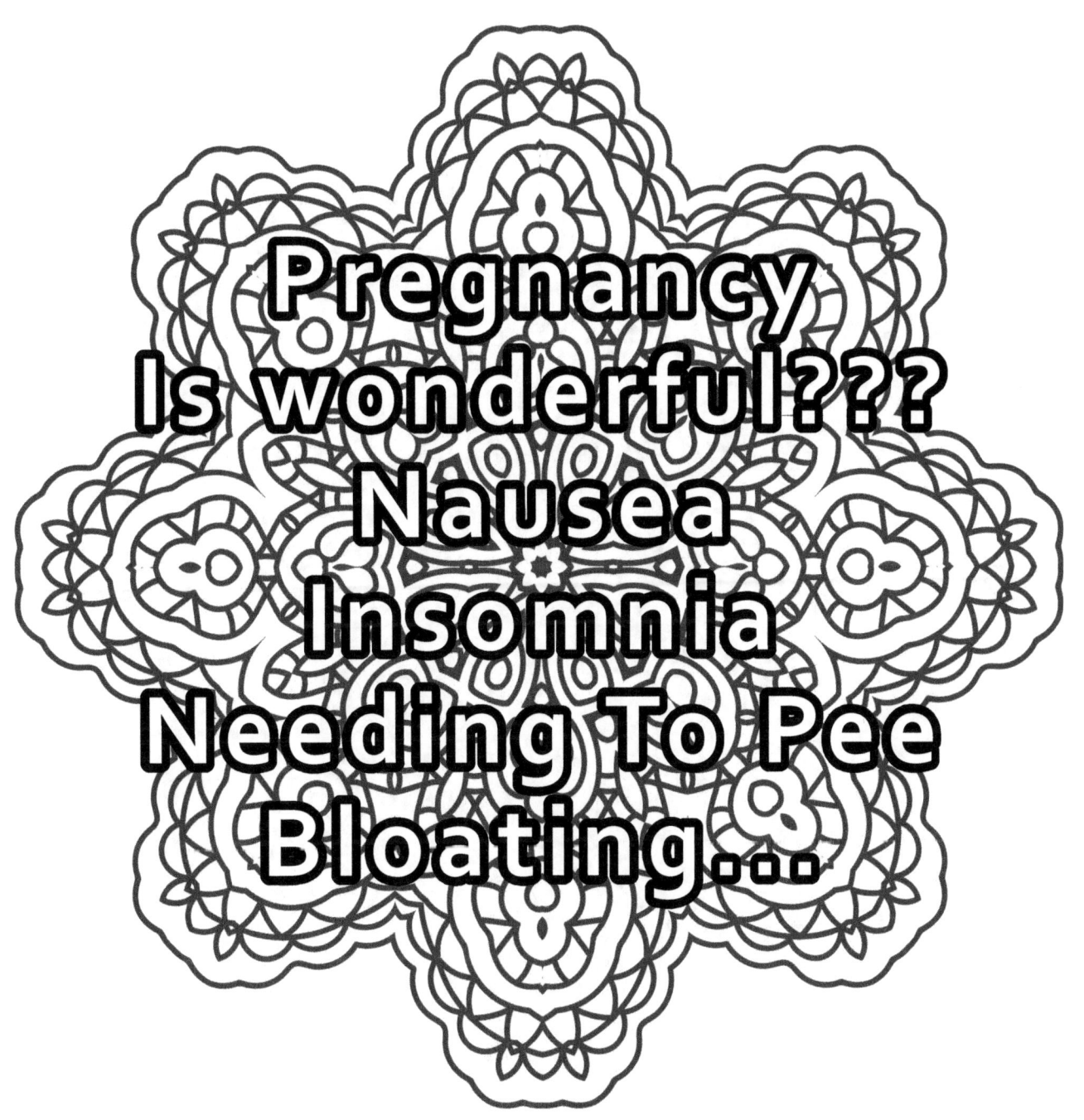

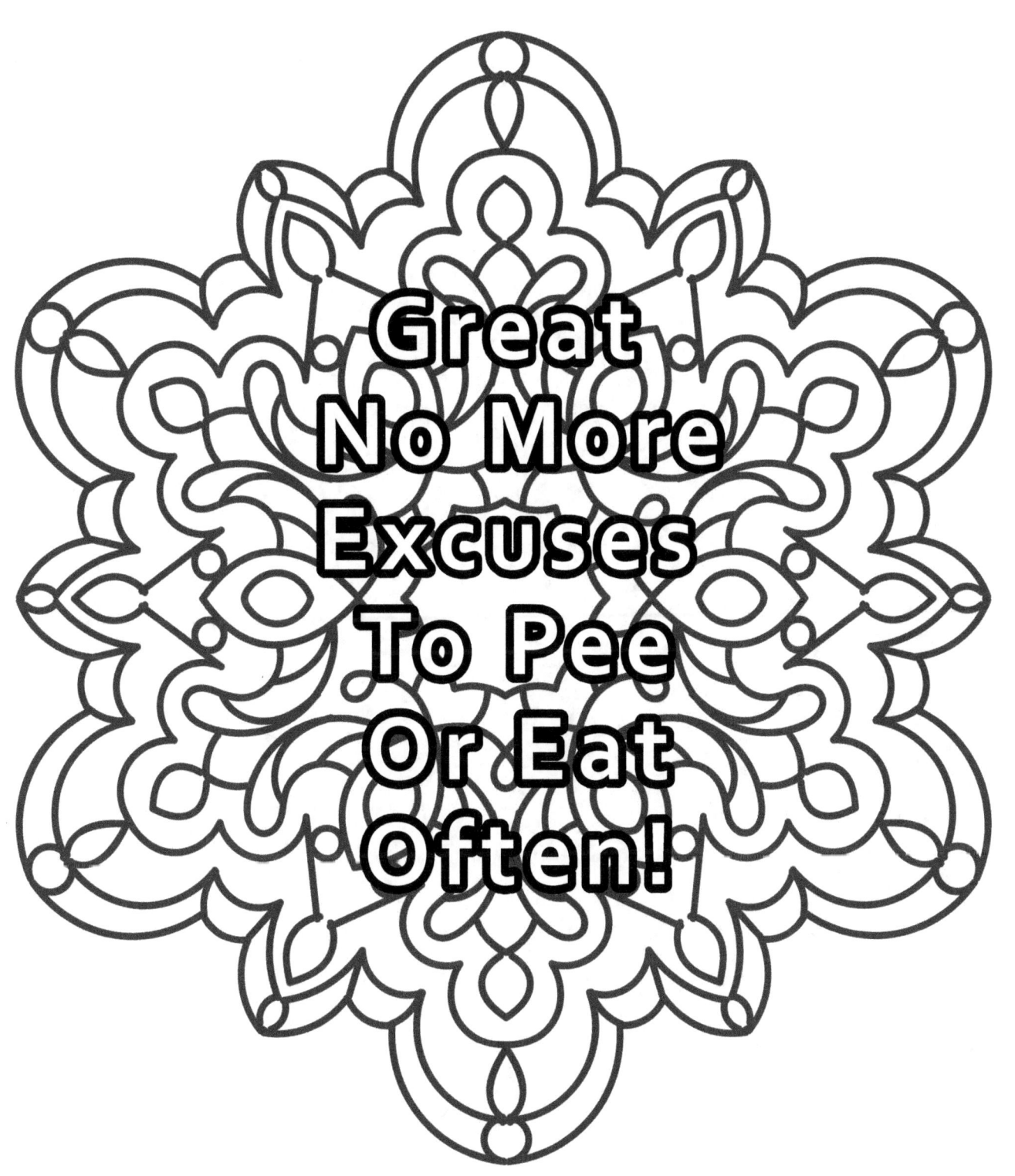

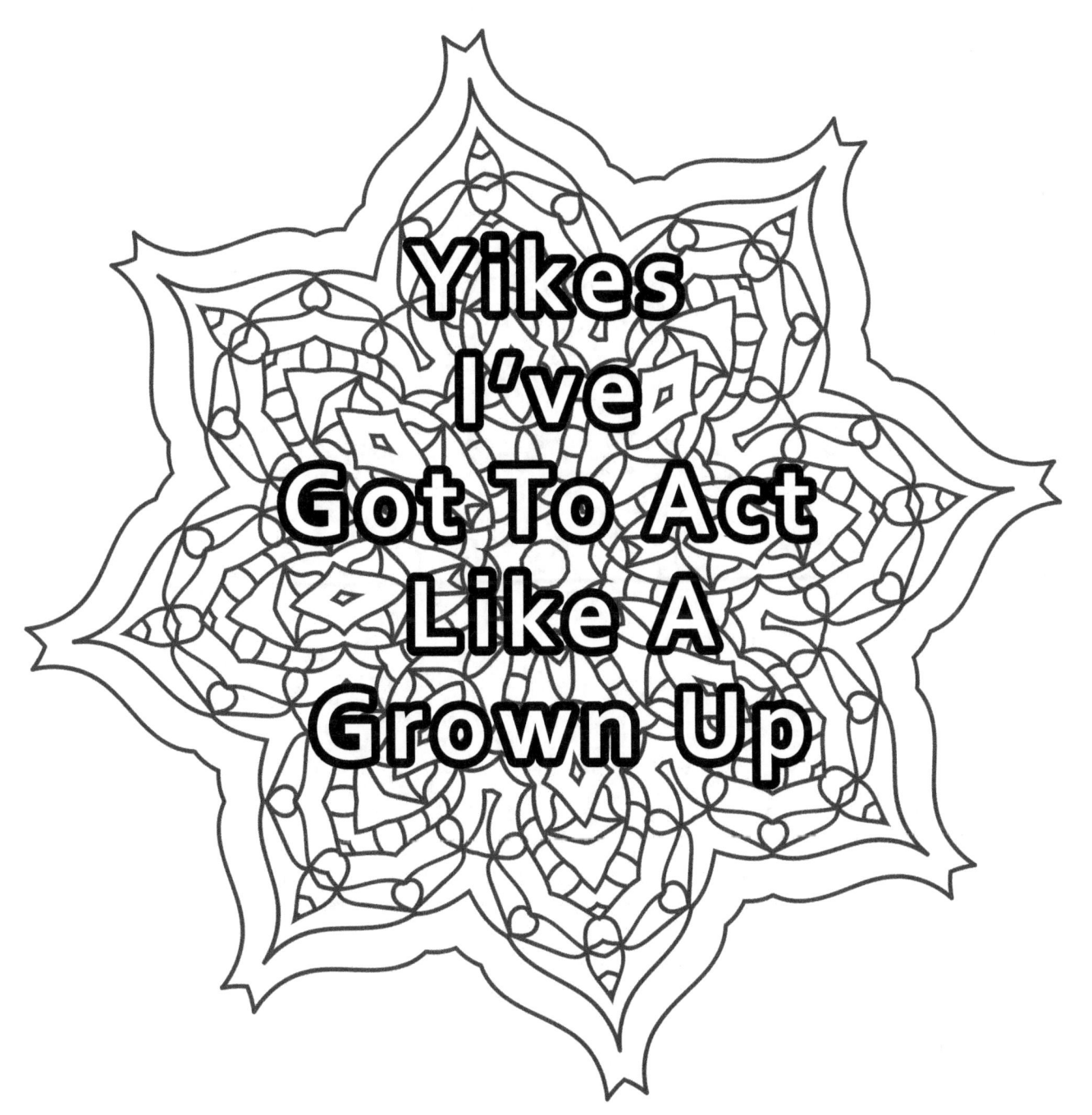

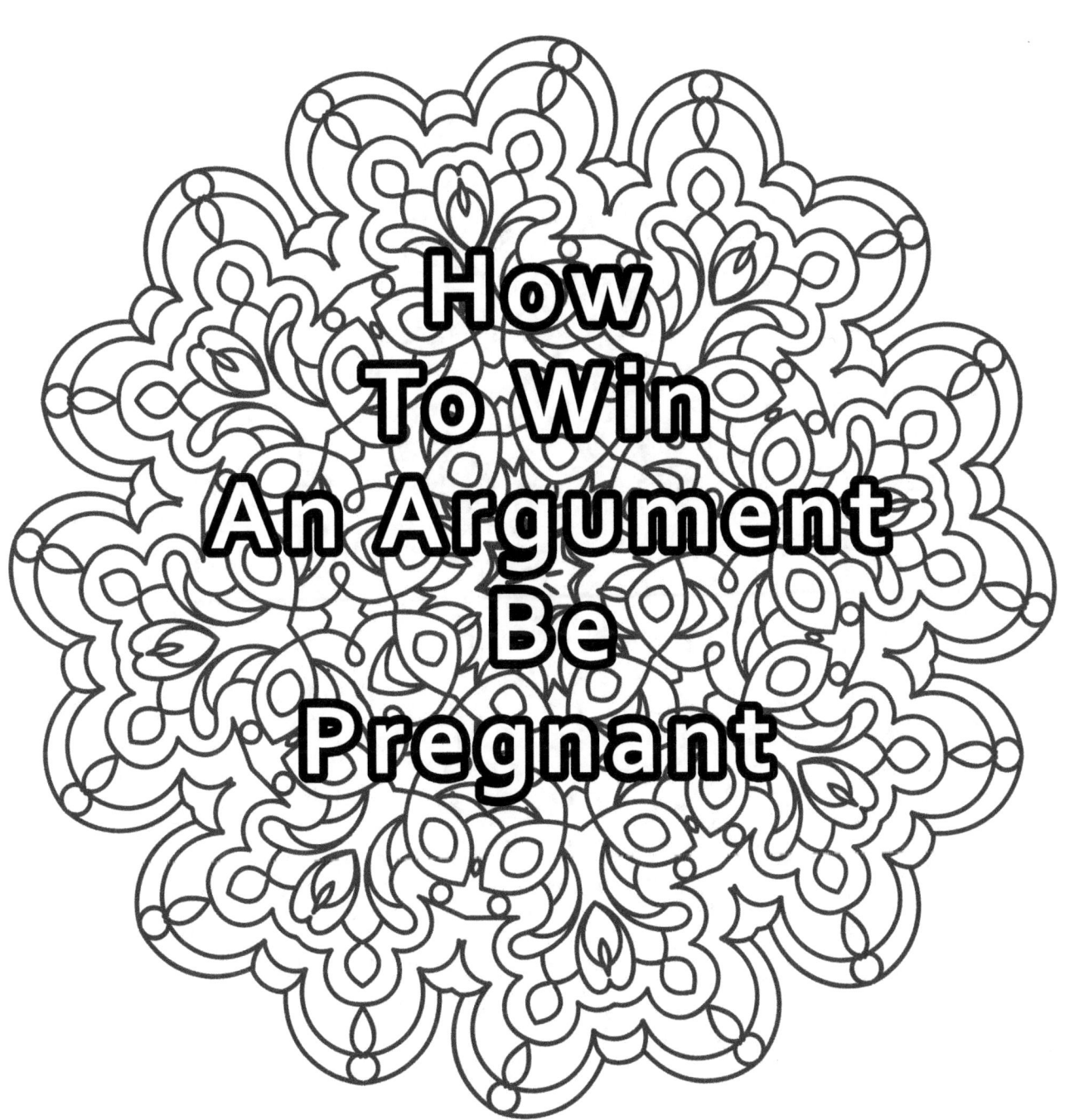

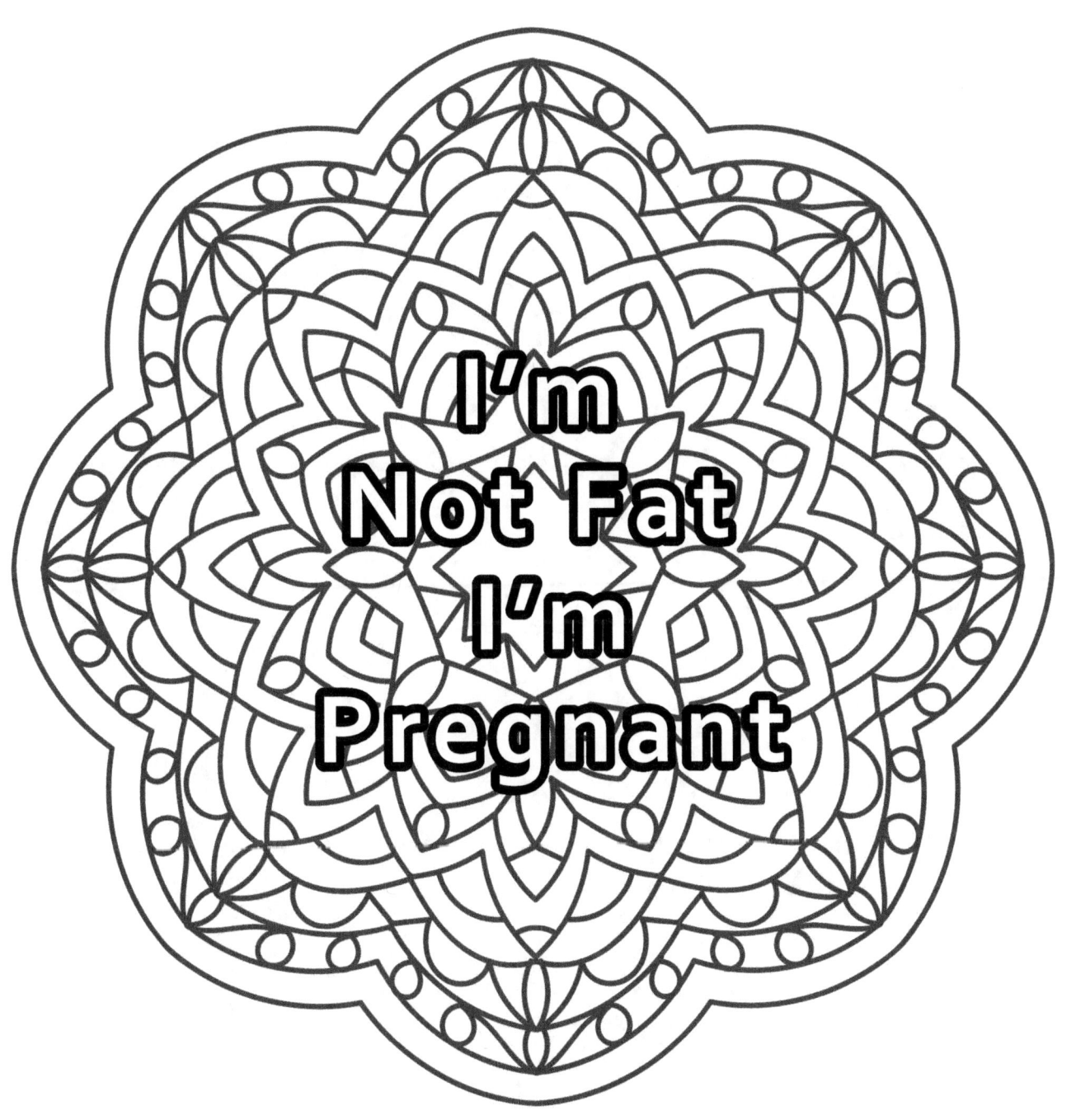

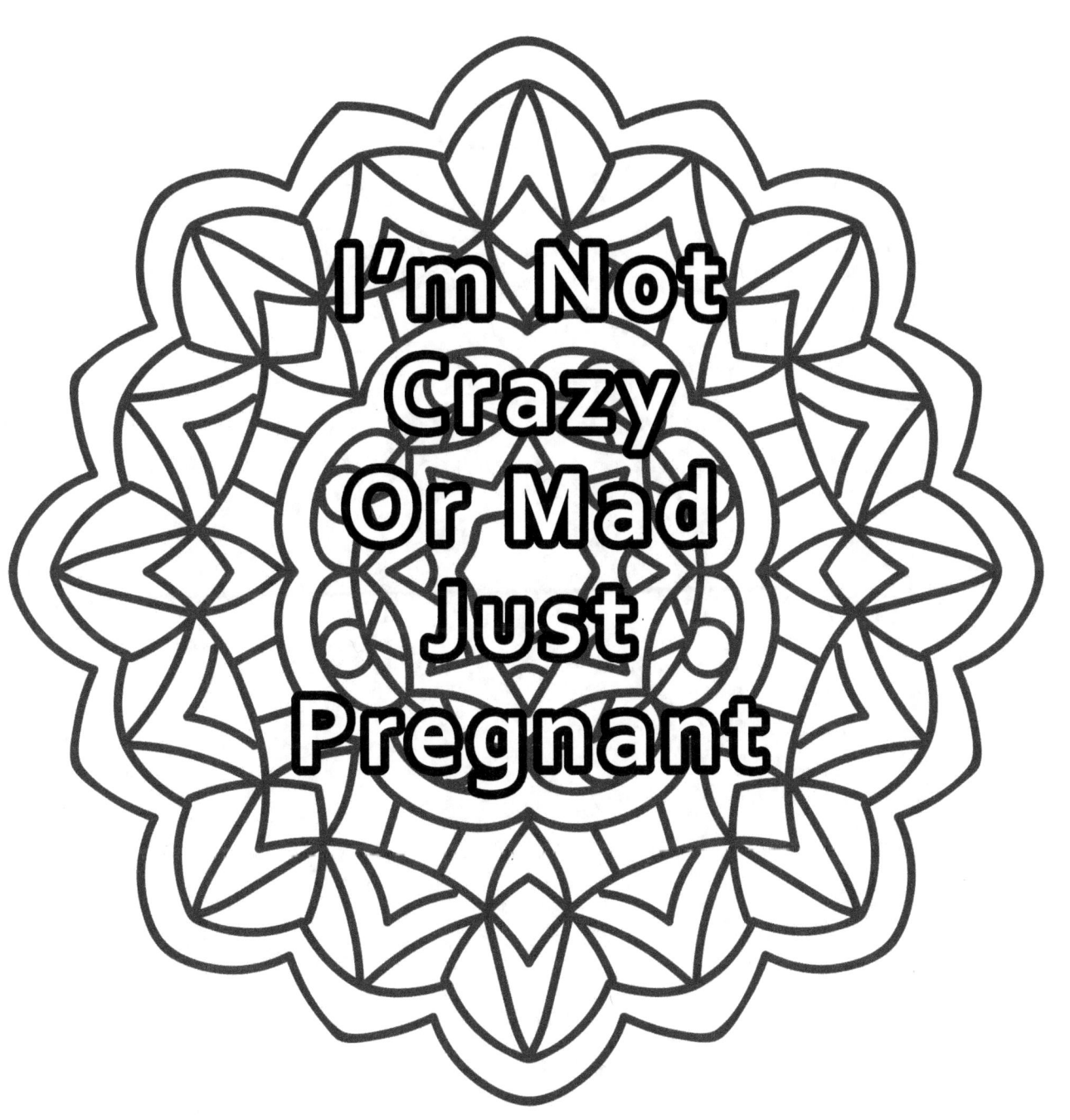

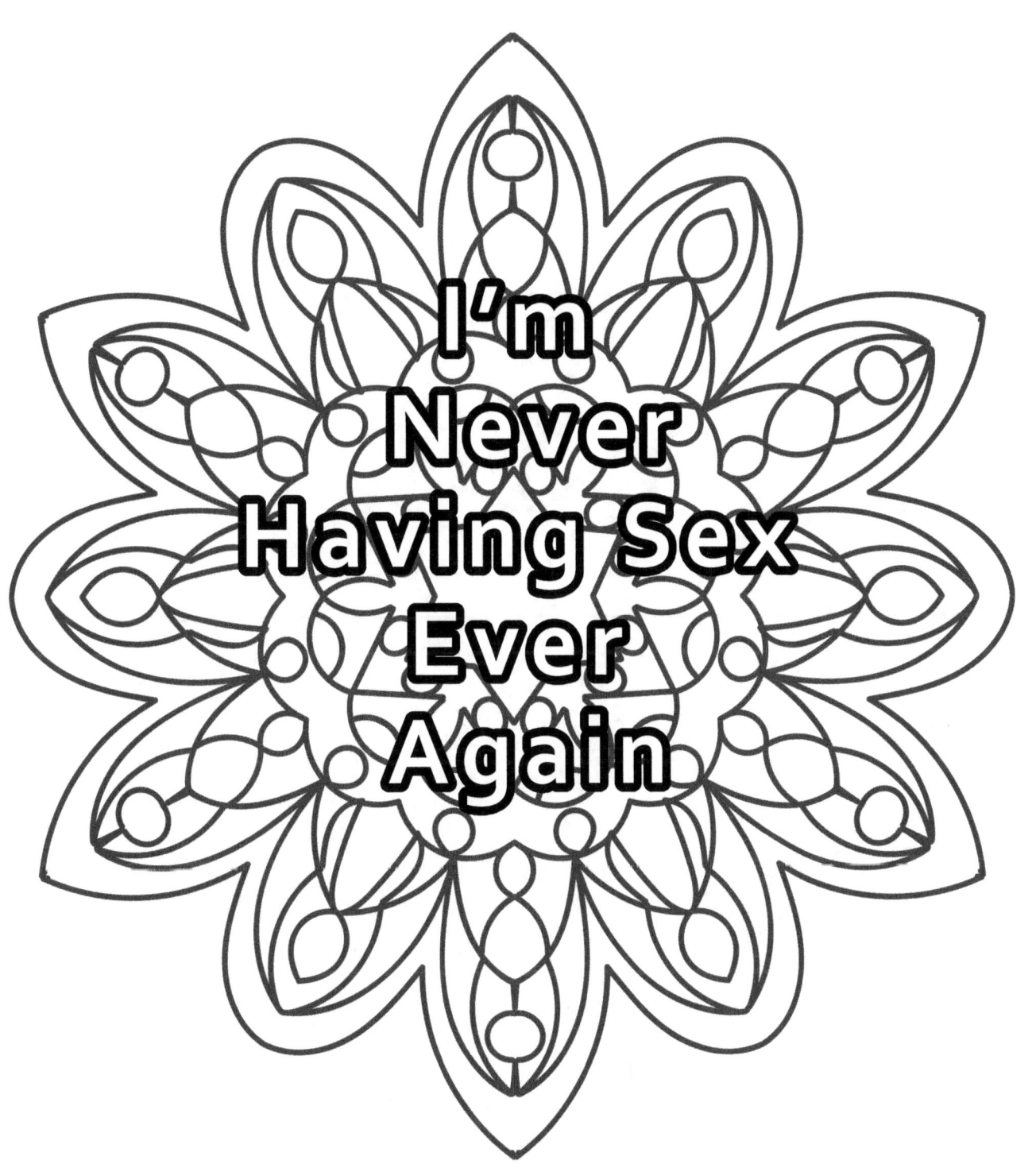

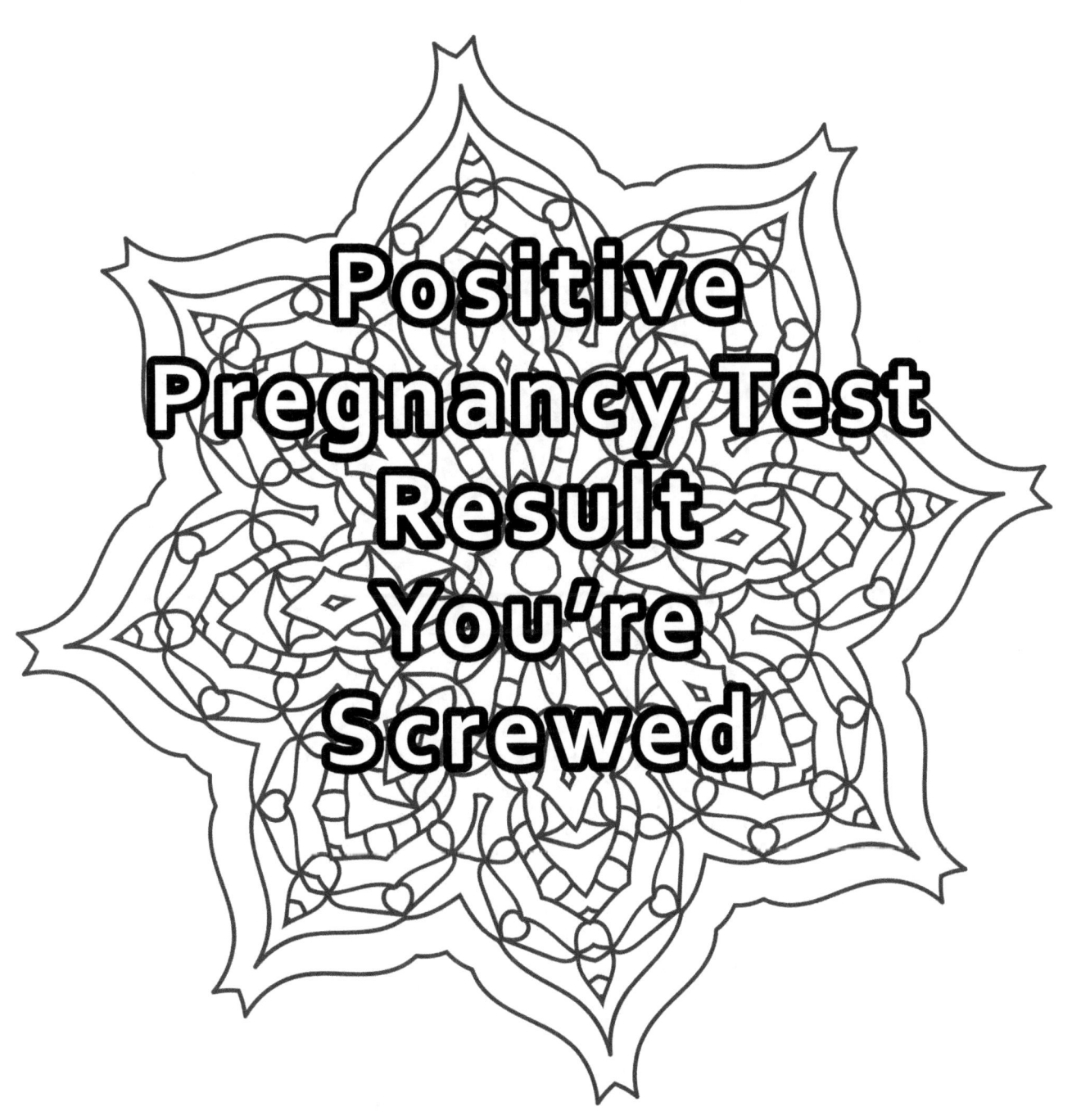

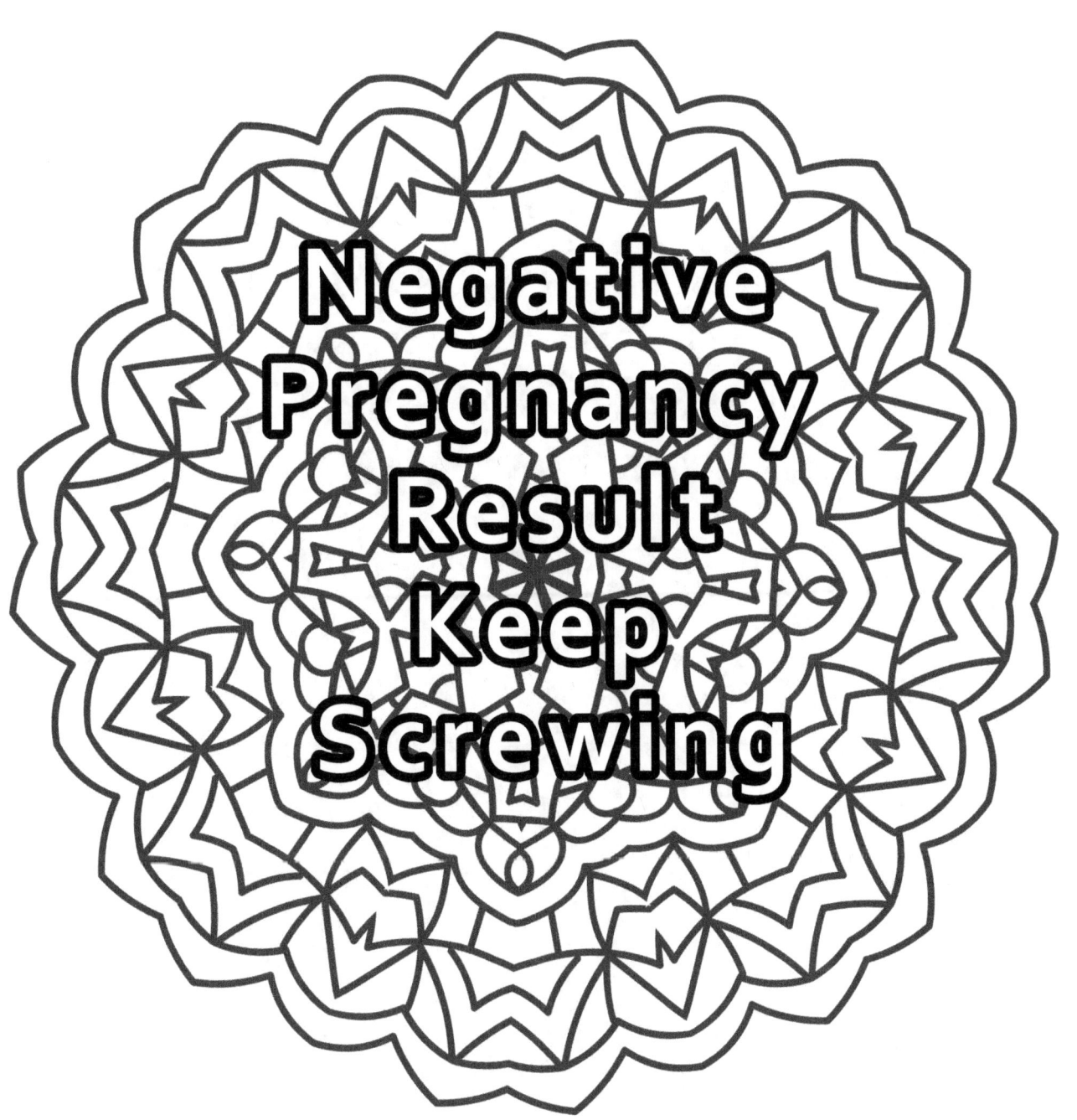

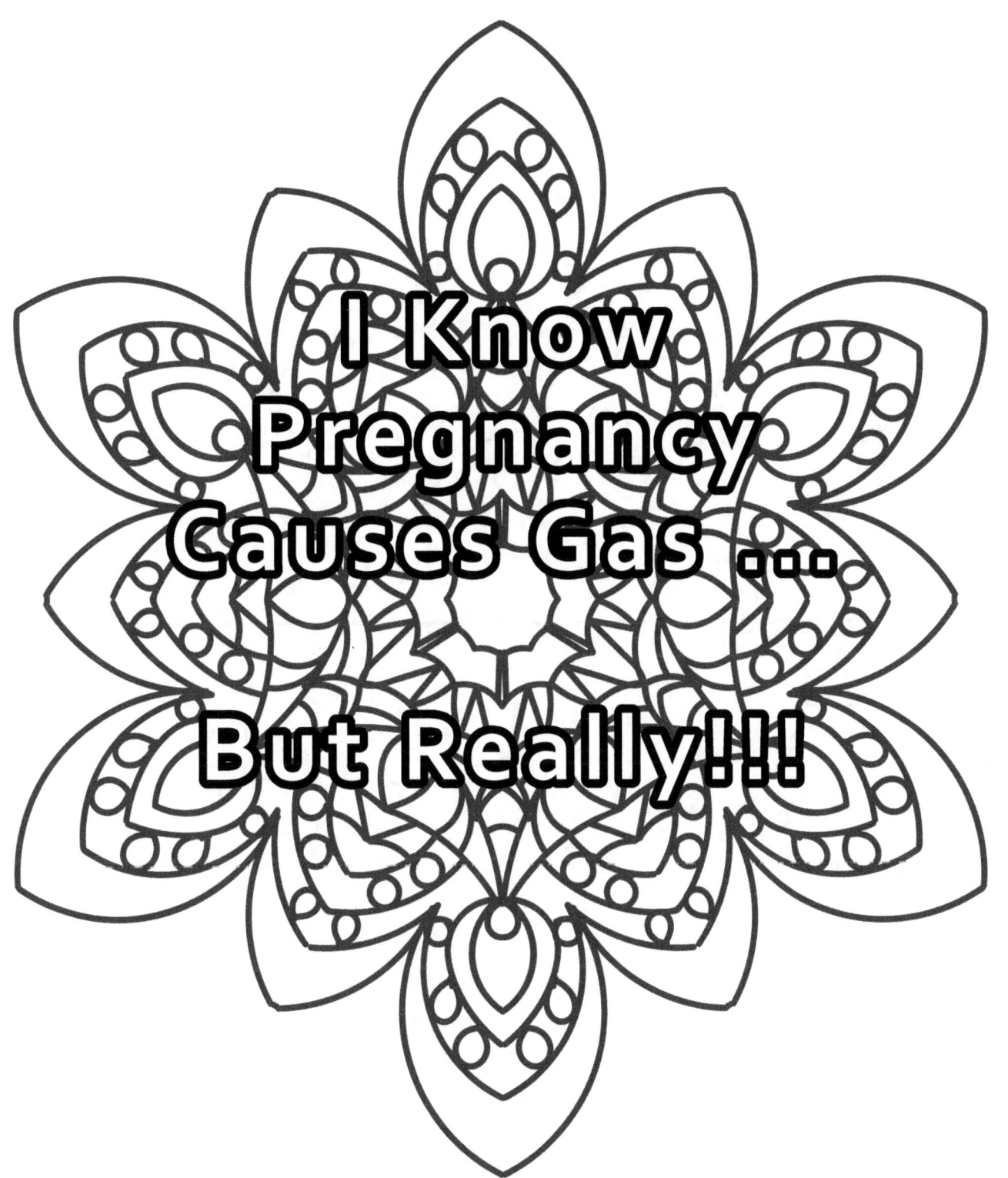

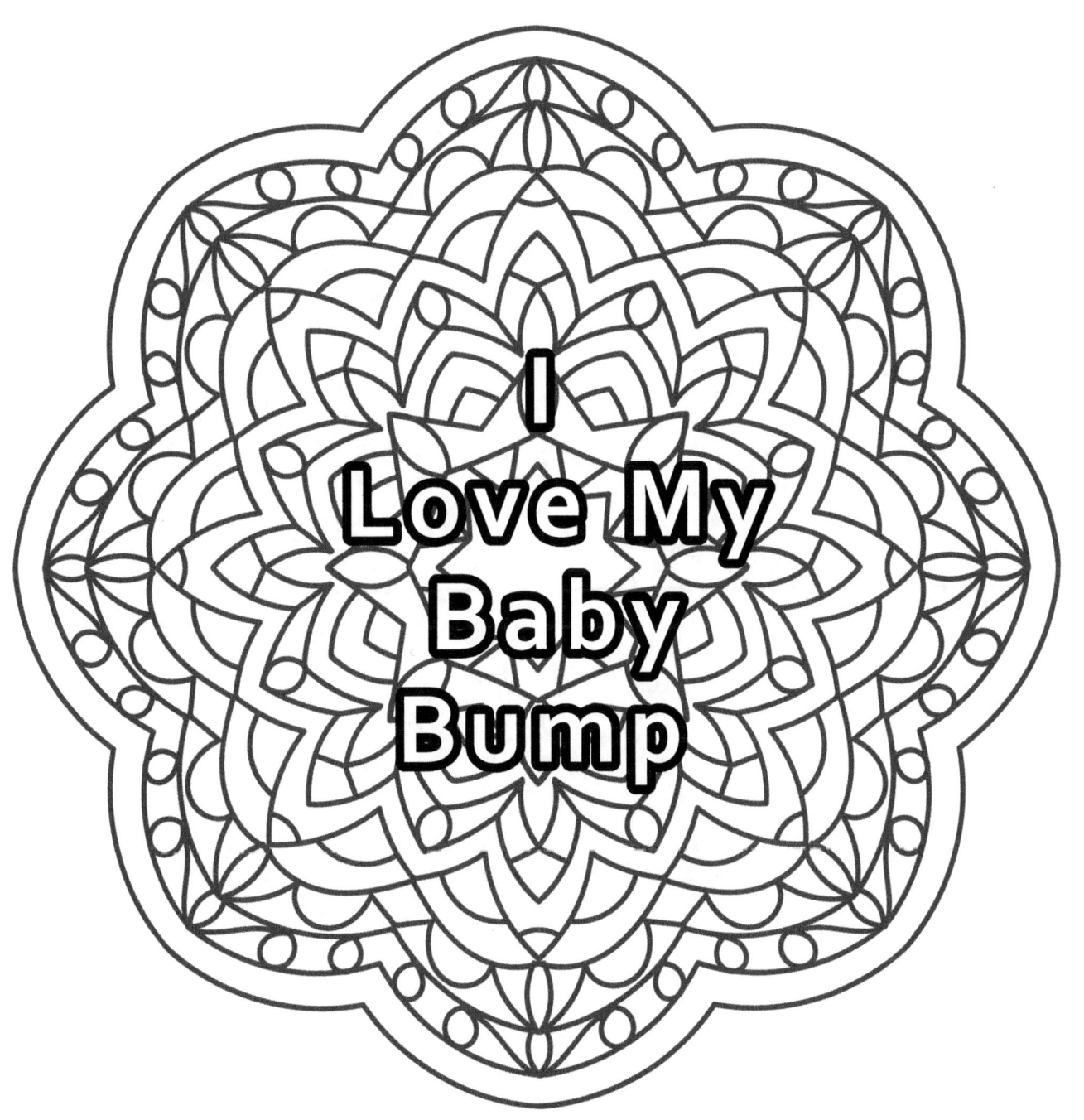

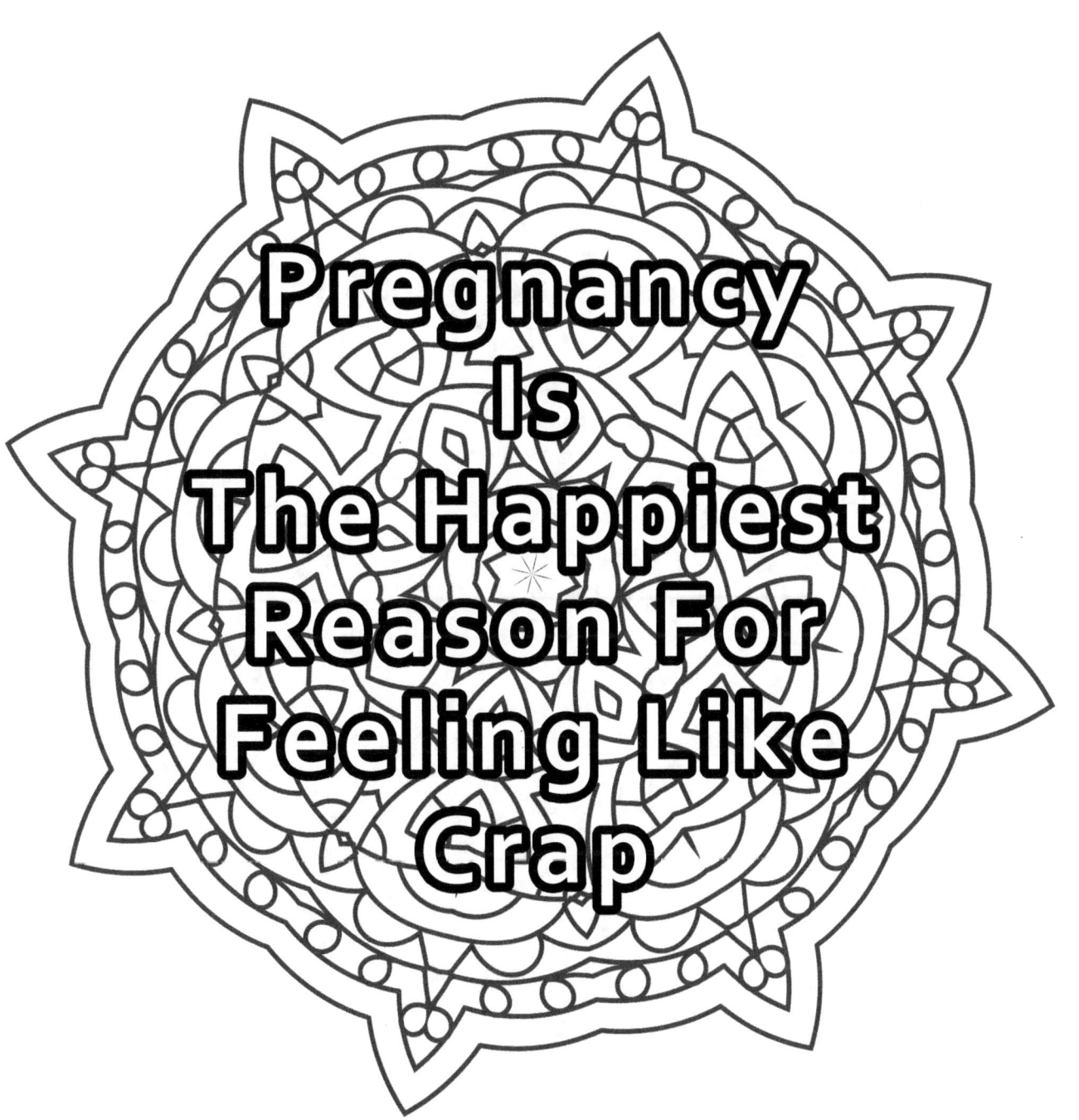

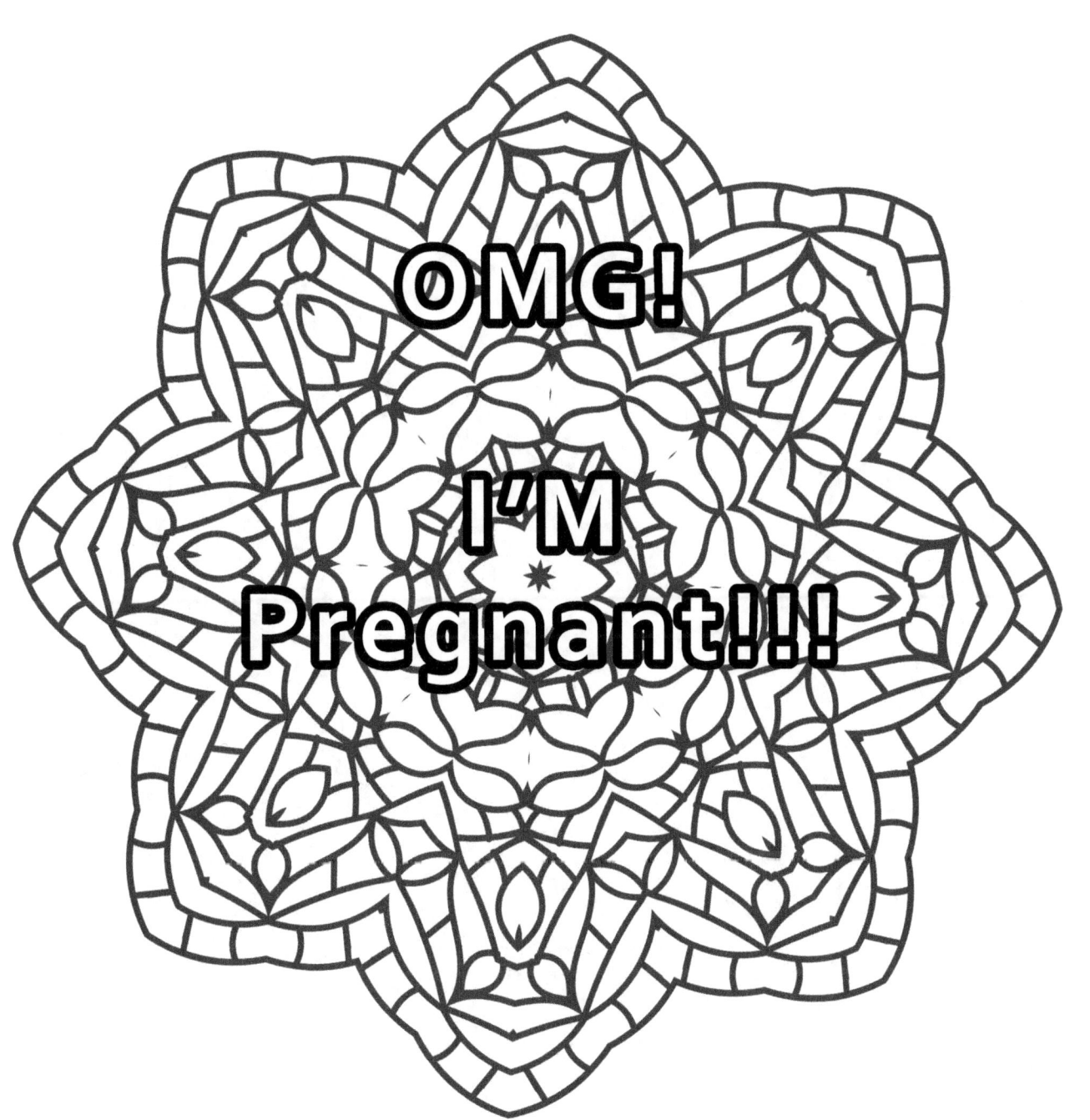

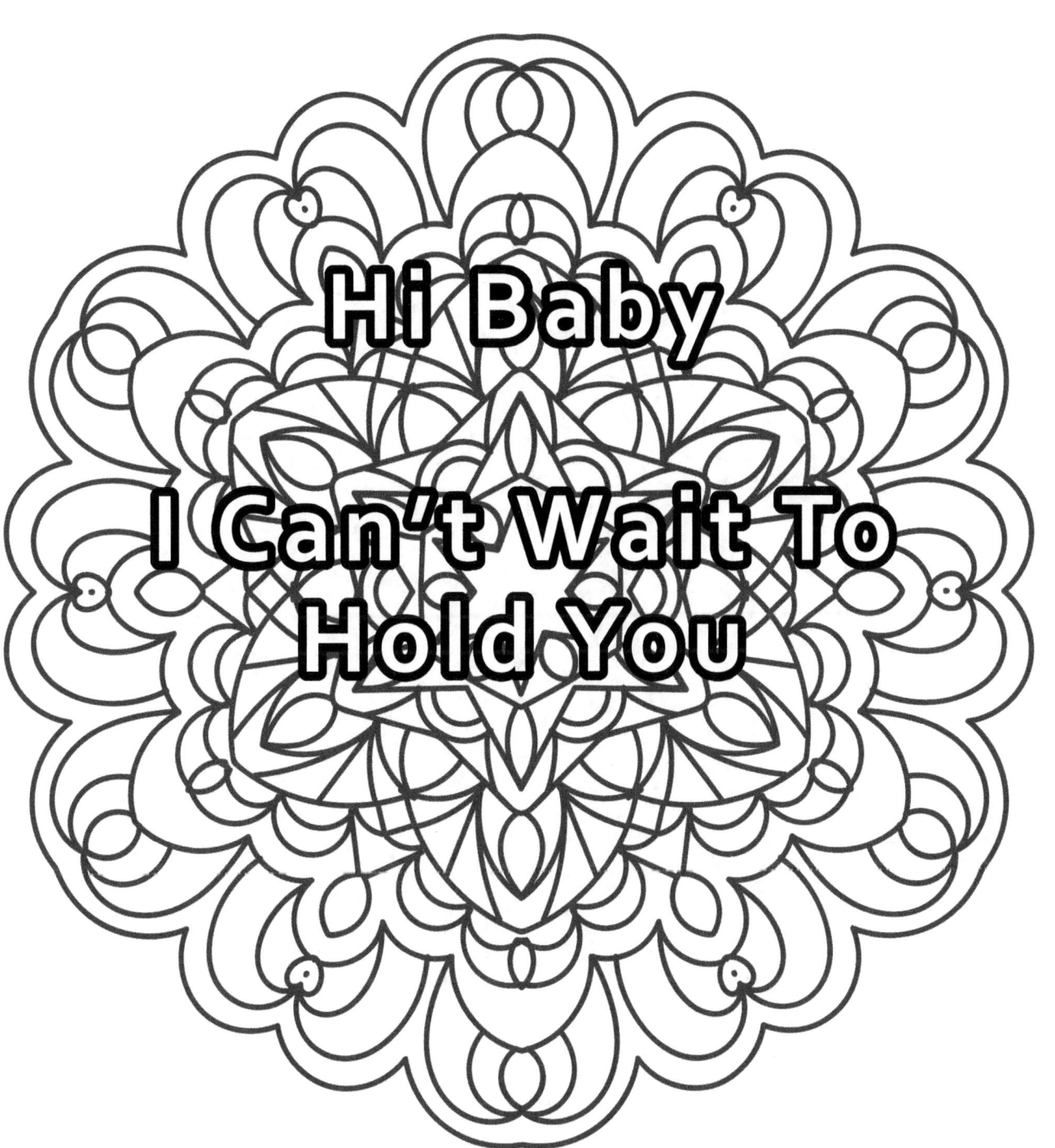

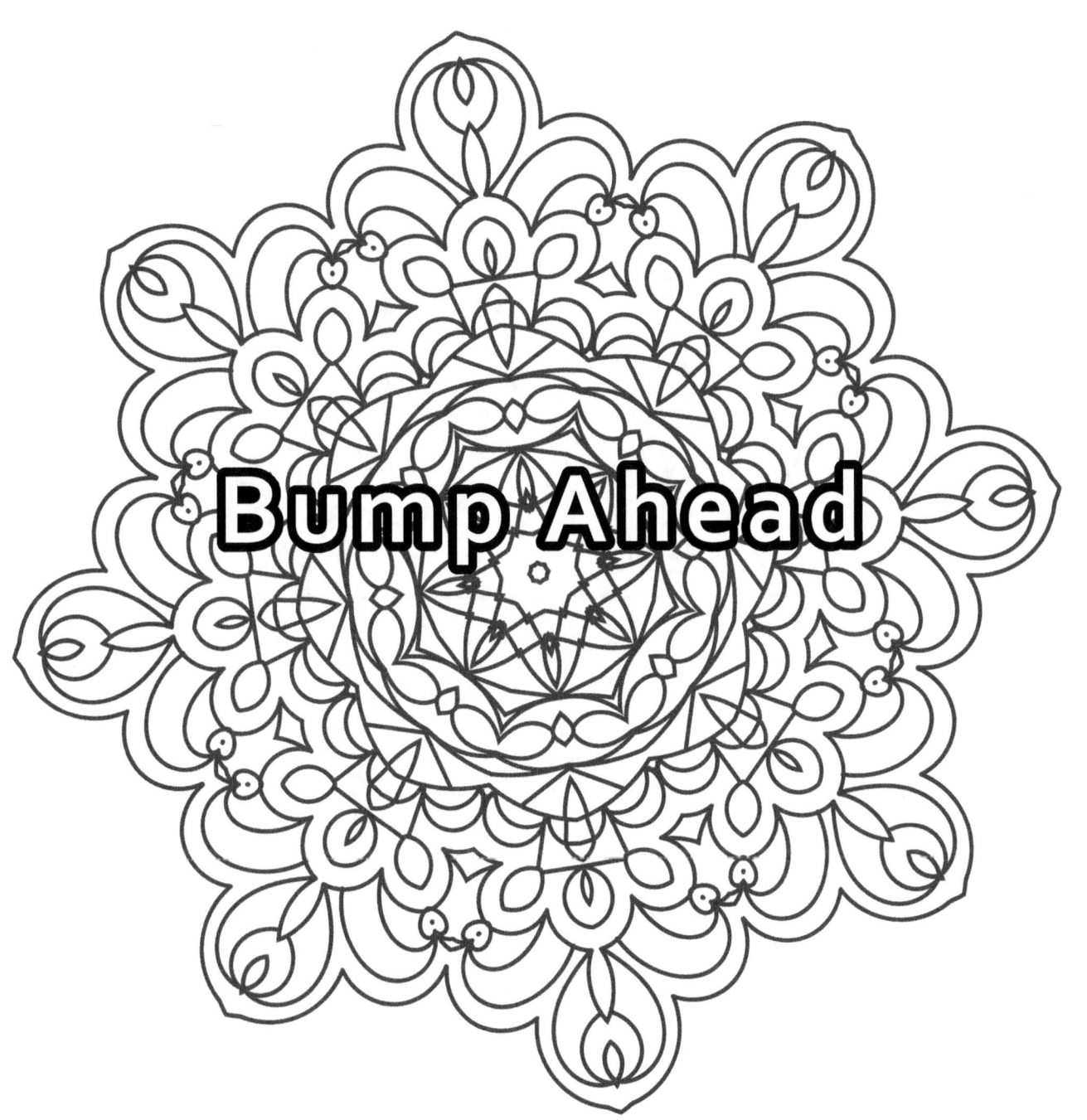

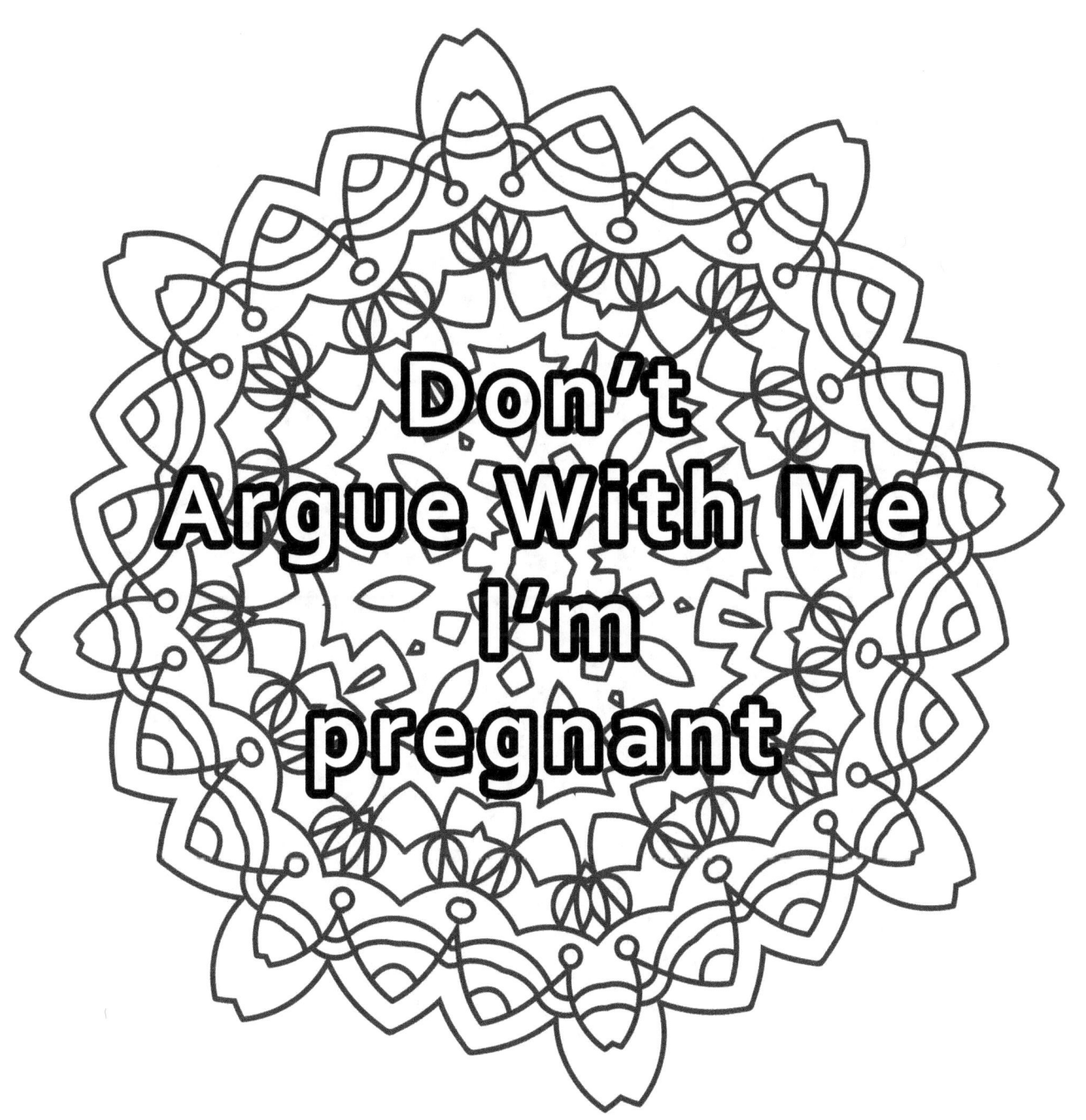

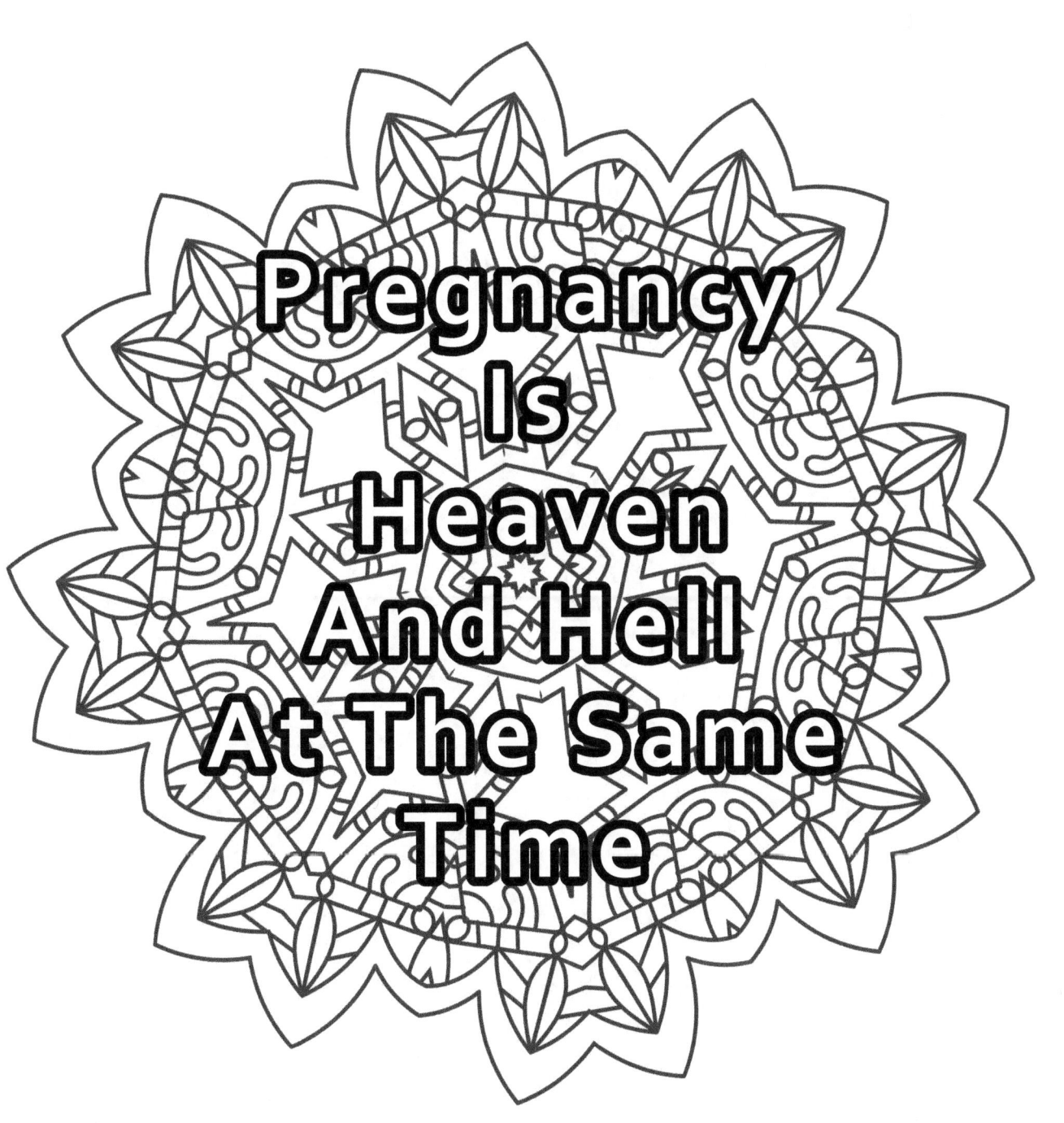

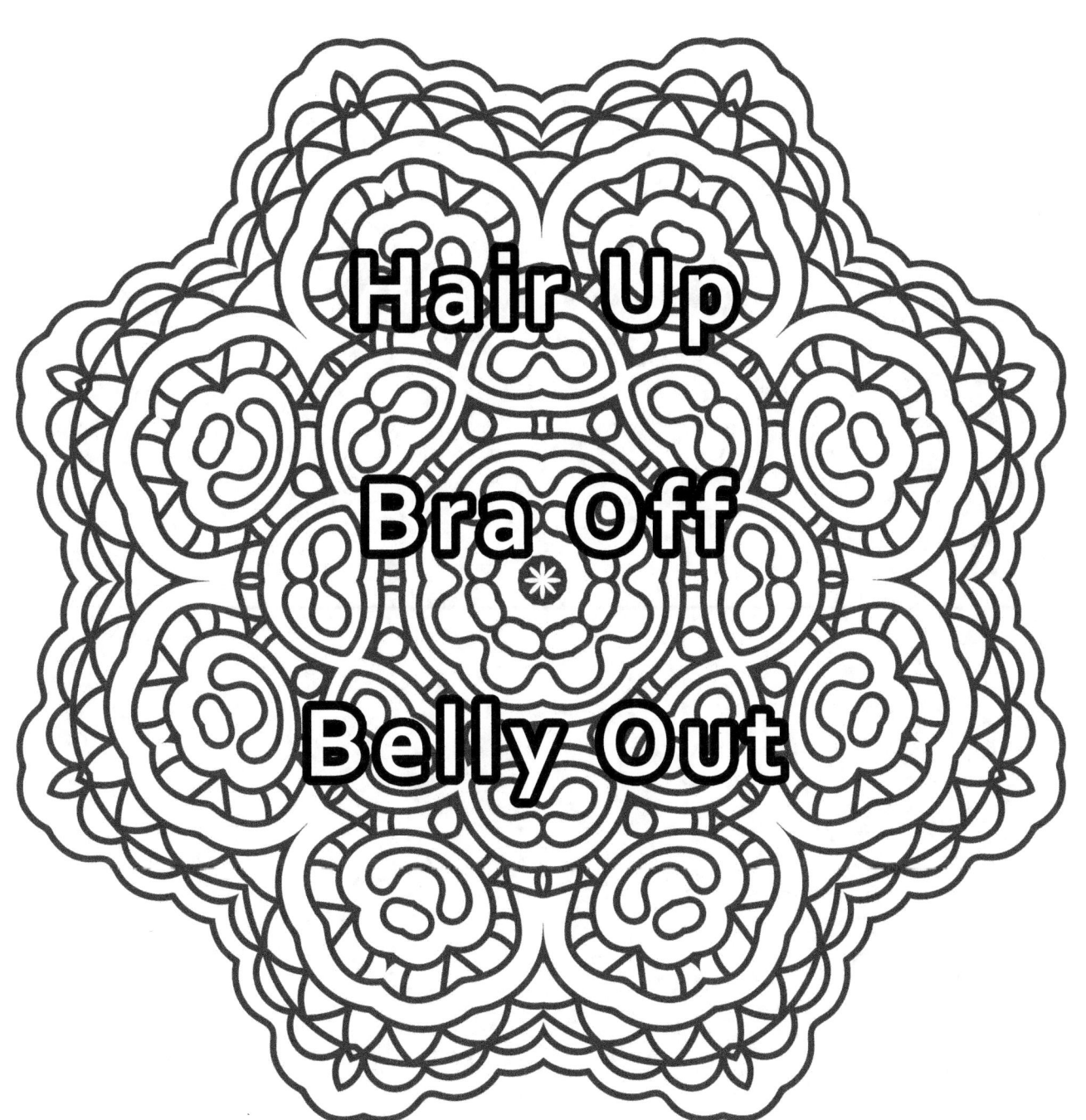

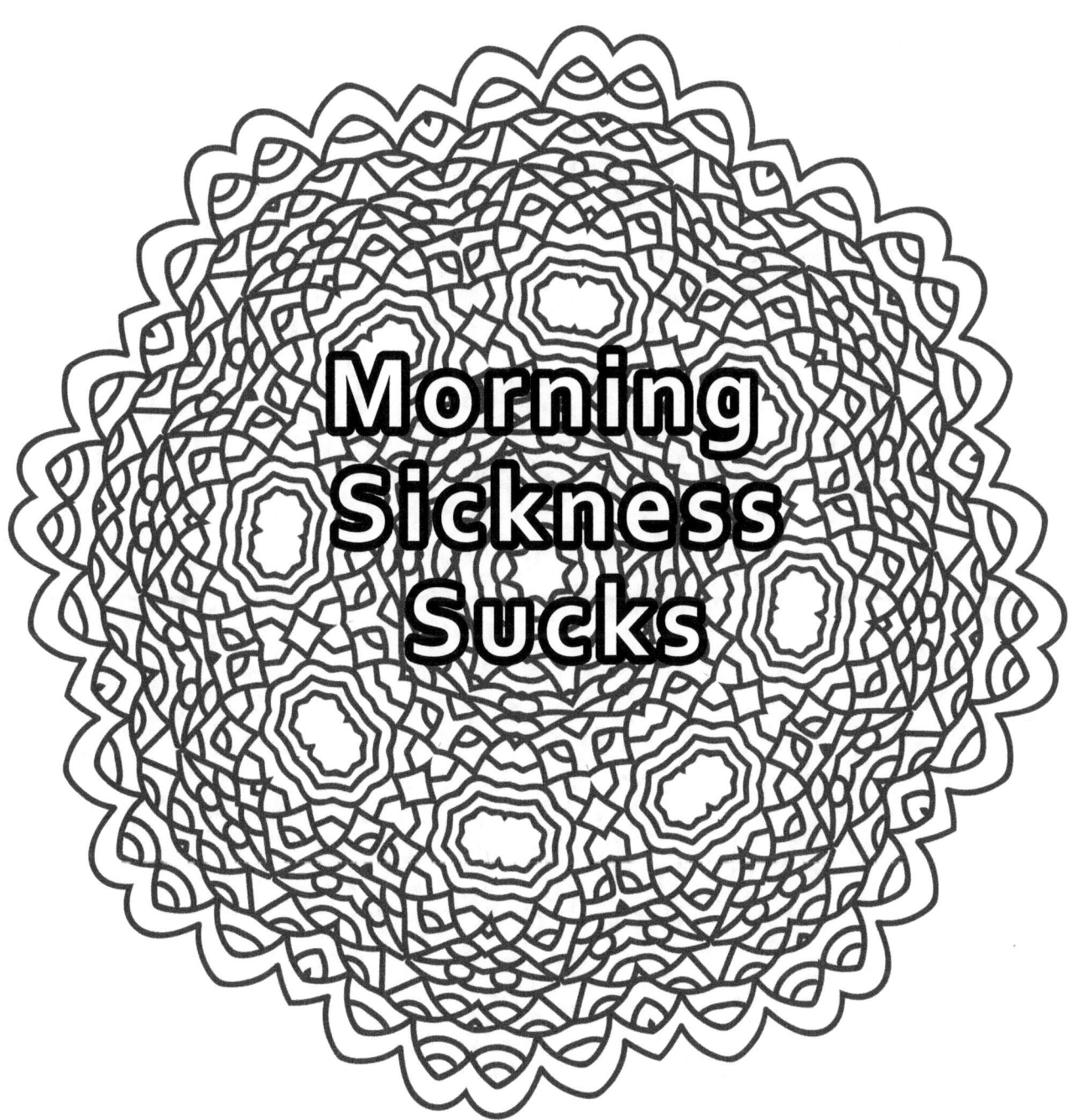

COLOR TEST PAGE

www.ingramcontent.com/pod-product-compliance
Lightning Source LLC
Chambersburg PA
CBHW062127220526
45471CB00010B/3910